From Multiple Sports To Multiple Sclerosis

FIGHTING THE MS BATTLE

(AN ATHLETE'S STORY)

Neil Hutton

Former athlete, coach, IT Consultant

Current father, grandfather, sports camp director, minister, writer

Future law student and retiree

Library of Congress Cataloging-in-Publication Data

Hutton Neil
From Multiple Sports To Multiple Sclerosis/Neil Hutton

IISBN: 1468134019
ISBN: 9781468134018
First Edition, 2011

Lenox Avenue Publishing
244 5th Avenue
Suite 2911
New York, NY 10001
212-252-2654
info@lenoxavenuepublishing.com
www.lenoxavenuepublishing.com

DEDICATION

I have so many people to thank for getting me to this point in my life.

First, I would like to dedicate this book to my mother, Betty, who passed away at the early age of 53 from complications with diabetes and high blood pressure. She was the nicest and most gentle person that I knew in the world. She was a favorite to my daughters and would not raise a finger or voice to harm anyone. Just the threat of her telling my father about an occurrence of something bad, was enough to keep us straight. I miss her heart and her voice.

The second person on the list is my wife Beverly. She had promised to be by my side when we were married, and promises to see me through all of the stages of life whether good or bad, until death do us part. Our roles have changed over the years and she has taken every role change in stride without missing a beat. She has nursed me through the heart surgery and the daily MS regime without wavering. God will continue to bless her and everything she puts her hand to do.

The third is my late grandmother Dora Sheppard. She probably left me the greatest gift she could and that was to pass away on my birthday. Now that day has real meaning to me. We nursed her from her death bed to health, to live out her last few years of life. It was tough to see her pass, but now she is in a better place with no pain or suffering.

The fourth is my complete family from my departed grandparents to our own grandkids. They were and are great treasures and gifts from God. Everyone is aware of my condition, but no one probably ever thought it could happen to the family's top athlete. But they are always there to support and to treat me the same.

TABLE OF CONTENTS

THE REALIZATION

On January 31st in 2001, I was positively diagnosed and officially notified that I had Multiple Sclerosis. I went to the University of Pennsylvania Medical Center for my second visit with Dr. Dennis Kolson to review the findings of all of my tests that were conducted during the previous eight months. With the test results and the history that I supplied him with months before, the diagnosis was not what I expected.

I expected to hear that my herniated discs were causing the trouble in my right leg, and that my blood pressure was causing my dizziness and vision problems, and that a pinched nerve in my neck was causing problems with control in my right hand. Never for a moment did I really believe MS was a possibility. I never even personally knew anyone with MS.

The only serious disability that I had personal experience with was Cerebral Palsy. One of my best friends, Gary has been confined to a wheelchair almost all of his life. He has always been an inspiration to me because he never let the disease take away his life. We played games together as kids, we talked sports endlessly, we went to opposing high schools and our schools were rivals in athletics. Gary was always the team manager because he couldn't walk. We always talked on the phone or visited when we were home from college. It was fascinating that Gary left home upon graduation from high school and attended Southern Illinois University. After his graduation from there, Gary went to California to live, work and play. He taught school, bowled, played and coached wheelchair football despite limited use of his arms and hands. He stopped playing when he said the game got too rough. The wheelchairs had gotten too fast and players would purposely try to knock the wheelchairs over.

Imagine that. Is that competition or insanity?

But the one thing that impressed me most is that Gary never let the disease take away his mind or his spirit. That is a hero to me. It's not the guy with all of the talent and athletic ability. It's not the guy with all of the smarts or intellect. It's not the guy who can run the fastest, jump the highest, score the most points, lift the most weights, win the most Oscars, or gets the most election votes. It is the guy, who survives when the world is stacked against him, physically, socially, culturally, and emotionally, who never quits and is willing to get the most out of his life, each and every day. He now includes me in the list of disabled African Americans. Believe it or not, I feel that it is an honor, not a curse.

MY BACKGROUND

I grew up as an athlete. I thought that sports were the most important thing in life. The one advantage that I had over most of the other athletes was that I was also a very good student. I was a straight A student almost all the way through elementary and middle school. I understood the importance of education and would not be denied the opportunity to learn. The competitive drive that sports gave me, I transferred into the classroom. In middle and high school, as far as I was concerned, no other boys in my classes would get grades as good as I would. I didn't really care about the girls. I thought they were smart anyway and they didn't do all of the sports stuff that I did, so I gave them credit for having grades better than mine. That was a lot coming from a skinny little kid with glasses, who was always one of the smallest in the class and also the quietest.

I can remember getting angry with the older guys in Burlington on the basketball court because I was young and small, and was not ever chosen to play with them. It probably didn't help that I had moved from Burlington to Westampton when I was in the third grade, and I wouldn't see my old friends until the weekends. My friends would eventually be allowed to play with the older guys because they went to school with them and the older players could see their development. In my mind, I was almost, if not just as good as them because I could dribble, play defense and play smart. I failed to realize that these older guys were in high school and I was still in elementary school or junior high, so the difference in size, speed, and skill was significant and it mattered in order to remain winners on the court.

Baseball, my best sport, was different. After floundering through my first year in organized sports in the minor little league, at the age of 7, with a mediocre team, I went to a championship team, the Detroit Tigers, coached by Mr. Carnivale and Mr. Fillipine. My father also joined as an assistant coach. He always took care of his boys. This was the beginning of a six-year stint where I began to show my dominance as an athlete.

First of all, size did not matter in baseball. It required good hand-eye coordination, a good throwing arm, and a lack of fear of the baseball. I was never afraid of anything dealing with a sport. That led to my being a baseball catcher for the next five years as well as a third baseman and pitcher. I was the guy with the "heat" and "the long ball hitter", as they call it in baseball terms. Having a really good throwing arm was a requirement for playing these three positions well. I wore number 24 because Willie Mays was my idol, until I grew out of that jersey. Then I wore number 12 because I said that if I was half as good as Willie Mays, I could play for the Phillies. We won 5 straight championships during my time with Mr. Carnivale, who by the way, was ahead of his time in coaching baseball.

During the time I played major little league baseball in Burlington, I had established myself as a basketball player in junior high school in Westampton. I was becoming a very good, if not dominant player in various sports. Whenever and whatever we played, I was always the first or second pick for any games. But as good an athlete that I was, I never, ever said anything to that fact. I was always a team player and was willing to do whatever it took to win. I was a quiet and humble athlete letting my play do all of the talking for me. For me, that was the only way to perform. Also, I wasn't as confident as people thought I was. You could never tell that by watching me play, but it was the drive in me that would not let my lack of confidence show. The groundwork was set for the rest of my life.

I was personally able to take a backseat when performing in sports or any activities. I left the lead role for anyone equipped to handle it. Playing the support role was sufficient for me as long as the final mission was accomplished. If I had to step up my role when needed, I was confident and driven enough to do it for the duration necessary and then slide back to my normal position. I didn't seek the limelight at any time because it wasn't necessary for my pride or ego. I understood the bottom line and despised not reaching it. I kept the emotion and stress of all of this bottled up inside for many years. That may have contributed to my blood pressure always registering as borderline hypertension.

MY SIBLINGS

Who says that having a lot of brothers and sisters is not fun? I didn't have a lot of them and I would have welcomed more. There were four boys and two girls in my family: Darryl, Mark, Timmy, Carla, Lisa and myself.

My oldest brother Darryl died before I was born. He would have probably been the best athlete of all. See, my dad was a fantastic athlete with a desire to play professional football. My mother was a hidden athlete who had skills but would never participate with us. My grandfather and uncle were athletes. The term local legend sometimes surfaces when hearing stories of all of their athletic exploits. So Darryl couldn't help but being a good athlete, although no pressure was ever put on any of us to succeed athletically. All we received was unending support and personal instruction if we asked for it. As it turned out, Lisa was probably the best pure athlete of all. I was probably the most driven.

But the thing that I liked the most was that we were all athletes. We competed against each other everyday and every season from sunrise to bedtime. We were used to turning on the outside spotlights until the wee hours of the morning to finish our games. And it wasn't just us. My cousins would come to the house regularly and during the summers, or we would go into Burlington and just play sports. The summers were fantastic. Playing basketball, football, strikeout, horseshoes, tetherball, checkers, cards, swimming, trampoline jumping until the cows came home. If you can name it, we did it. Competition? You bet. Fierce? We knew no other way. That is one of the reasons why the spotlights were so critical. Losers didn't want to end as losers so new games would start again. We had to put a cap on the number of games in a series to stop from playing all night. We all honed our skills right at my house. Did this competitive fire pay off? It certainly did for me. Why? I am the one fighting MS.

HIGH SCHOOL

High school is where I first started playing organized football. My father, being a former football player, didn't think it was necessary for us to play before then. He knew we were good athletes and I don't think he wanted our bodies to begin receiving punishment any earlier than necessary. I didn't agree then, but I am glad that I didn't play before high school. All that I missed were a few touchdowns and pats on the back, or maybe a broken arm or leg. None of it was necessary. I would get enough of that later; the good and the bad. I always said that if I had a son, I would not let him play football until high school. Like father, like son.

I didn't get much playing time as a freshman. I was the third smallest guy on the team and I was a quarterback. I had always been a leader by example and quarterback seemed to be the right position for me. Besides, I had a good arm and I could run. That didn't really matter much. There were bigger guys who could do what I did at that level. I quarterbacked the 5th quarter team. Those were the guys who didn't play during the first four quarters. My freshman career wasn't very eventful, although I did start wearing contact lenses. I was ready to call it quits after the season and concentrate on basketball. I was small and never thought I would grow anyway. We didn't appear to have the tall genes in our family. My father and the varsity football coach, Mr. Gordon, talked me out of it and into playing one more year.

It was also during my freshman year that I began to get disenchanted with baseball. I was no longer pitching and playing third base, but playing centerfield like my idol, Willie Mays. But that wasn't enough for me. I wasn't really involved in the game playing centerfield. We had pretty good pitchers and very few batters hit the ball to centerfield. I was told that I was moved there because of my speed and versatility. To this day I never accepted that, although centerfielders are usually good athletes with good speed. In my case, there were other players who only played one position for almost their entire careers and to make room for them, the versatile player, like myself, is usually moved to fill another need. That has been my life story in and out of sports. I played one more year of baseball and then joined the track team in my junior year. That change was easy since I long jumped in gym class farther than the long jumpers on the track team.

Basketball was my favorite game. I was always quicker than most. Although shorter, I could jump higher that anyone else that was near my height. I was always the point guard who could really shoot, but very rarely shot much in a game unless we were playing Burlington, Bordentown or Palmyra. That was because I knew the players personally and played against them outside of school and they knew what I could do. I had to show them that I could still play although the role on my team was different than what they were used to seeing. I was the ultimate team player in high school and made sure that our main scorers got the ball. But I was a defensive stopper. It was always a challenge for me to stop the opposing scoring guard. It is the sport that I enjoyed playing the most and gave me the most exercise.

But a funny thing happened during my sophomore year in high school. I began to grow. I was becoming a normal size guy. I was no longer shorter than the girls. I used to be so short that they would take off their shoes to dance with me. How embarrassing! With that increase in height, came an increase in confidence. It was probably not apparent to anyone else; only to me. Because of that, the possibility of playing sports at the college level became real to me. I didn't know the level at which I could compete, but I knew there was a level for my playing ability.

THE EPISODES

When I was a junior in high school, I joined the track team. I was always a very quick runner but never had the stamina for the longer distances. The 100 yard dash was really too long for me, but the 40, 50, and 60 yard dash were perfect. The problem is that those distances aren't run outdoors and I didn't run indoor track: I played basketball. As a result, my main events were mainly the jumping events; the long jump and high jump and sometimes the 100 yd. dash and the 440 yd. relay. I ran the hurdles one time in a meet, in the second heat, and took third overall without practicing. That would have probably been my best running event, but I didn't pursue that. Jumping was my specialty and although the hurdles combined the two, I don't know why I didn't continue it. They say that hindsight is 20/20.

One day when we were running 100 yd. dash trials in practice to see who would be in the first and second heats of the track meet, something unusual happened. I was always the third fastest runner in the 100, and expected things to turn out like they always have, but on this day my legs felt unusually heavy like they were water logged. I mentioned to Coach Ridgway that something was wrong with my legs but I didn't know what, but that I would run anyway. Needless to say, I got beat by a guy that I had always beaten before. The rest of the practice was very sluggish. I could not jump well at all. My legs seemed to be dragging all the time. I had no idea what was going on, but I did not think it was serious enough to pursue.

I can remember having sporadic days like that before but they weren't important because I wasn't in competition and I just worked right through it when it happened. Each time, the next day I was fine. As for the track meet the next day, I ran in the second heat and won it and my time was faster than the guy who beat me the day before and ran in the first heat. Things were back to normal.

I had grown primed for competition. Adversity was always just another obstacle to overcome. If necessary, I would push my body past what I thought was normal into an area that could only be sustained with adrenaline and an internal source of strength. My competitive drive kept me pushing on.

When I was in college playing football at Penn State, we would sometimes have to practice on the astro-turf if the weather was bad or the ground was covered with ice or snow. Multiple times I can remember working out with "heavy legs". The same sensation that I had in high school would manifest itself while practicing. I didn't recall the sensation before practice, only during and after practice. As during previous occurrences, I would push myself through them to finish my workouts. Because I was usually one of the fastest runners on the team, I could work through the episodes and no one could really tell the battle that I was having.

One episode occurred on a day when the pro scouts were timing the players in the 40 yd. dash. They were really just concerned about the upperclassman in preparation for the NFL draft. It's a good thing. I was an underclassman and my time which was usually extraordinary, compared to the rest of the team, was just an ordinary time. It didn't hurt me personally because I was an underclassman.

During all of these bouts with "heavy legs", I never believed that anything was really wrong. I just passed it off saying that my ankles got taped too tight for practice, or that I thought I might have a slight circulation problem in my legs due to the turf, or shoes, or something else external not internal. A possible circulation problem should have been enough to have it checked. But I didn't. I believed that I was a superbly conditioned athlete.

The physical issues that I had in college didn't appear major and never stopped me from playing. I got injured just like everyone else. I had the normal muscle pulls, busted fingers and sprains like everyone else. I had shoulder surgery for a dislocation after my sophomore year, torn cartilage in my knee, a separated collar bone, but nothing that stopped me from missing more than one or two games except for the surgery.

The surgery forced me to medical redshirt the 1975 season and to make perhaps my most important and regrettable decision regarding football. I always viewed myself as an offensive player, skill wise and personality wise. The two go hand-in-hand. Defensive players are more reactionary and aggressive, and offensive players are more precise and calculating. Although I performed well defensively, I enjoyed running and catching the football much more. I wanted the opponent to attempt to stop me, instead of the other way around. Defense brought on stress, but offense was natural and instinctive.

After meeting with Joe Paterno before the start of spring football, he told me that I would be the #1 running back on offense or the #1 cornerback on defense. The decision was mine to make. He gave the pro and cons of both and even considered my future after Penn State. In the end, I decided to forego my dream and switch to defense for the good of the team. I did it once again. I knew that we could always get a running back, but getting fast cornerbacks with man to man coverage skills could be difficult. That was my most regrettable decision. There I was again, sacrificing for the good of the team.

After switching from running back to cornerback, I played well enough to get drafted in the ninth round by the New York Jets in 1978. I didn't really dream of playing in the NFL because football wasn't my favorite or best sport, and I wasn't playing the position that I felt I really should have been playing. I knew that I would get drafted because of my physical ability and speed. I also played in the Japan Bowl All Star game and the player personnel director from the Jets was on the trip.

In rookie camp, Bobby Jackson and I were the top two cornerbacks and we both went into the pre-season camp looking to start. But in camp my passion for the game died, mainly because of the politics involved in the NFL. It was a business and the fun was gone. I couldn't accept that, so I left camp and went on the voluntary retired list. The next year I got traded to the Washington Redskins, got hurt in preseason camp and later placed on waivers. My NFL career ended there and I have no regrets. I knew I had the ability to play in the NFL and that was enough for me, but I didn't really have the desire to play out of position. Life goes on.

In 1984, I accidently received the opportunity to go to football camp with the Philadelphia Stars by doing a favor for my old coach, John Rosenberg. He asked me to help him coach at a free-agent camp at Veteran's Stadium. While there he asked me to workout, resulting in an injury to my Achilles tendon. Although I wasn't in top shape, I performed well enough to be asked to attend the preseason camp in Florida. I decided to attend although I was still slightly injured. After a few days there, I knew my career was over and after staying down in Georgia with my cousin for a few days, I came home, emptied of the professional playing baggage.

Because I loved basketball so much, I would use it to stay conditioned for every other sport and began coaching it at the high school level. Although the skills required were different, it gave me the basic conditioning that I needed; running, jumping, changing direction, quickness, agility, stamina, and the list goes on. When I turned 30 years old (critical to athletes), I stated that I would never stop playing basketball because I loved it and it kept me in shape. I was looking forward to competing in the over 30 and over 40 leagues because I was still competing against the younger players and quite successfully. My body and mind always seemed younger in age than it actually was in years.

Then something happened. I remember playing basketball with the guys from the church in the early 1990's and for some reason; I had trouble controlling the ball when I dribbled. It used to be that my hands always felt like they were part of the ball when I dribbled. This day my hands felt foreign to the ball. It was almost like I was slapping at the ball. My hands felt numb and I couldn't feel the ball like I used to. So to get around this, I would let someone else bring the ball up the court and when I got it, I would pass right away or shoot it. It didn't effect by defense, only my offense. This feeling never went away and I never told anyone. I just began playing less and less, and coaching more and more. The numbness was in my hands and feet, but it never really registered that something was really wrong. It was all a part of early denial. It also didn't help that I was really beginning to feel the effects of my football-damaged knees. When I would strain them, it would take months to recover instead of days. I was not used to that. I was a superbly conditioned athlete. I thought it would all eventually go away.

Finally, in my mid-30's, I stopped playing basketball completely. Giving up football and baseball weren't very hard for me. They weren't my favorite sports and they required special skills that continually had to be worked on, but putting away basketball was difficult. Many times I would see my friends competing and something inside would try to get me to step onto the court. But the realization that things physically were not the same would keep me off of it. I was too much of an athlete to be embarrassed in competition. I had to make sure that I was never dressed to play basketball and never kept a set of playing clothes in the car, to ensure that I stayed off of the court.

I finally asked God to remove that fierce competitive desire in sports from me so that I could be at peace with my decisions. He honored that request and from that point on, just watching or coaching sports became a real enjoyment and satisfaction enough. Ironically, I made that request during the time when spiritual growth became an important part of my life. I had learned that I couldn't just rely on acquired knowledge, experience, and myself over the years, or any other person, but that there was a power greater than any man; and that power was in Jesus Christ, the Son of God.

THE BIG ONES

In the spring of 1992, while working as a consultant at PECO, I noticed that I was beginning to have sporadic balance and vision problems. As a result, I scheduled an eye exam to replace my contact lenses and began wearing my glasses.

The project that I was working on was a top priority company project and the programming that we were performing was very unique and time consuming. The magnitude of the effort caused many a sleepless night trying to figure out the logic behind our programming intentions. It was one of the most intense projects that I had been associated with. Anxiety and stress were results of the scheduled demanding tasks. I thought that this was the cause of my not feeling well.

When I went for my eye exam, my blood pressure was taken before anything else was done. The eye doctor was shocked at the results and retook my pressure. It continued to disturb him. He asked who my primary doctor was and immediately called him to relay the results of my blood pressure. I was told to go straight to the hospital in Mt. Holly to have it rechecked and monitored. To this day, I still don't know what the reading was.

At the hospital I was given medication and monitored for the next few hours to see if the pressure would lower. It eventually did and I was released. The next day I had to visit my personal physician. After a thorough examination, he told me that my pressure was on the borderline high side and placed me on blood pressure medication to help lower it. This was the beginning of my fight against medicines.

I knew that I had been under a good deal of stress from work, but my blood pressure was only borderline high. After a couple of months, the balance and vision problems went away. All of these symptoms were attributed to my blood pressure, but now I am not so sure. It wasn't until I had a later episode, that I could account for what happened at PECO.

In April of 2000, while working as a consultant at an insurance company in Blue Bell, Pa, I noticed a problem with my right hand. The occurrence of the problem was so sporadic that initially I thought it was muscle cramps. While writing, I would suddenly lose the ability and coordination to form letters. I always write fast and messy being a programming consultant because the notes are just for me, and I thought that my hand was cramping because of the amount of writing that I was doing. I grabbed my hand, squeezed and massaged my fingers for about 10 seconds, and then they were okay. Initially this would not be a common occurrence during the workday but it would later become a daily occurrence. Then it became a multiple daily occurrence.

About the time of these occurrences, I began to have balance difficulty when rising from a seat and walking. It would take me several seconds to gather myself before walking, and then I had to make each step deliberate to keep from tilting to one side and walking a crooked line. I would have to be very careful going up and down the steps or stepping up on a curb. Because of my discipline, I would force myself to adapt and be very careful to hide any problems that I was having.

I also began having problems staying awake in the afternoon. This was happening every day after my lunch hour whether I ate lunch or not. Between 2:00 – 3:00 I would begin to have a difficult time concentrating and keeping my eyes open. I would get extremely tired and felt like I needed a nap to make it through the rest of the day. Needless to say, I would catch myself falling asleep at my desk for a few minutes because I couldn't control it. Several times I went to my car during lunchtime to take a short nap to combat the afternoon problem. It helped when I could go to sleep, except for the fact that I didn't want to get back up again.

Because of these episodes, I began to worry about my blood pressure again. I had stopped taking the blood pressure medication sometime after it was first prescribed in 1992. My blood pressure was always considered borderline hypertension since it first became a concern in my senior year of high school. I knew the dizziness that it would cause, because of my mother's situation with high blood pressure and my own. I also knew of the loss of sensitivity in my fingers that would occur if my pressure were high. This never happened much and I can recall the specific occurrences of it over many years. The first time was when I was holding a hot pan of baked chicken at the dinner table without potholders and didn't feel the heat of the pan. As a result, there were a lot of shocked eyes at the dinner table that evening. Those sensations lasted exactly one week and then everything was normal again. I missed one high school football game because of it. The other two times were once in college and once while working at Philadelphia National Bank. Each episode lasted exactly one week.

Also, I began having sporadic focusing problems with my eyes. I thought again that I was having contact lens problems. I only wore my glasses at home so I didn't realize the problem with my glasses. I then began wearing my glasses for a while to give my eyes a rest from the contacts. It helped a little, I think, but I still had clarity problems with distances. With all of this happening, my thoughts were on my blood pressure and the possibility of a stroke.

Things finally became critical at the end of April when I was attending the Penn Relays with my friend Dave Riley. We drove over to Philadelphia and parked a good distance from the stadium. It was a difficult walk for me not just due to my unsteadiness, but also because of my herniated disks. It made walking for more than a few minutes very difficult for my right leg. I would lose muscular control of my leg and my knee would begin snapping back as I walked. It forced me to limp and to begin dragging my right leg. I would fight through it as much as possible. Sitting down for a few minutes would restore the ability to walk but my desire was to always get to where I was going as soon as possible. Why prolong the agony if there was no pain involved? That was the surprising thing. It always looked like I was walking in pain but there was never any. The only discomfort was the soreness in my back and the snapping back of my knee.

After going into the stadium, my desire was to sit in one spot, eat my food and not go anywhere as long as possible. I did just that. Walking up the stadium steps was a chore and each step had to be deliberate in order to be safe and not fall. There weren't many people in the stands yet so I had a free path to where we were going to sit. Of course we sat up fairly high in order to adequately see everything. The relaxation was welcomed.

After sitting for several hours and enjoying the relays, the time came. We both had to go to the restroom. By this time, the stands had been filling and our row had many people on it. I immediately began thinking, 'How am I going to navigate this'? The only thing I could do is to follow Dave. He could clear the way for me. Meanwhile Dave didn't know about the problems that I was having except for the herniated disks and the difficulty walking sometimes. He didn't know anything else and I didn't tell him. He started down our row over the people and I followed him. But while I was stepping over feet, I lost my balance and fell onto a lady sitting on the row. I apologized to her, got up and finished the row but when I stepped into the aisle, I lost my balance again and fell into a sitting position on the step. I know that anyone watching me thought I was intoxicated. My coordination was like that of someone who had been drinking. The only thing I drank was fruit punch.

Dave never knew all of this was happening. He started down the steps and he thought that I was right behind him. I gathered myself, stood up and began walking down the steps. I made it down okay but the embarrassment of the falls was tough to handle.

We found the bathrooms, for me with some difficulty, and after exiting, stood in the tunnel speaking to people that we knew. I was having trouble focusing, thinking, remembering, talking, and balancing but as long as I was in one place, I could manage. When it was time to go up, I told Dave what happened. He was shocked. The first thing he said was: "Why didn't you call me to stop and help"? There was no way that I was going to call him with all the noise and people in the stands, and to bring more attention to my mishap as embarrassed as I was. If I could get up, I knew I could make it.

We went back up into the stands to see the rest of the relays. The people that were on our row were gone so it wasn't much problem getting back to our seats. There weren't specific seat assignments anyway. Now the only thing I had to be concerned about was walking back to the car after the relays were over. I tried to forget about that and just enjoy the relays. I am pretty good at that and that is just what I did. The worst was over. The stands would be fairly empty when we left and Dave knew the situation, so I wasn't really worried about leaving the stadium. I walked as fast as I could to get to the car. Wow!

TIME TO TELL

As bad as things were on the Saturday of the Penn Relays, I didn't say anything right away to anyone, including my wife Beverly. The first reason was that I very rarely went to the doctor because I always believed I would naturally recover from anything. I didn't like taking medicine, which is why I had stopped taking blood pressure medicine seven years before. The second reason was that Beverly had stopped working the previous year. Previously, we always carried our medical insurance through her employer since I became an independent consultant in 1985. I did not want to incur medical expenses that we would have to pay for if it weren't necessary. I knew that she would be going back to work soon anyway.

I took off from work on the following Monday and Tuesday. Before going to Bible study on Tuesday for a class that I was teaching, I casually mentioned to my brother, Timmy about the episode at the Penn Relays. Beverly heard the story and became extremely upset that I hadn't said anything. Timmy called the doctor's office (we all had the same primary care physician). Dr. Press asked to speak to me and he scheduled me to come in the next day for a checkup. That was the beginning of eight months of complete heart, blood, neurological, and MRI testing. That was four months of visits and testing that I would have to pay for. I thank God that I did not have to go into the hospital. We would never have been able to afford it. Beverly started working again in September.

Dr. Press immediately prescribed blood pressure medicine, which this time I decided that I would take until he released me from it, which would probably be never. Unless God performs a miracle, or it can be lowered through my diet, I will have to always take it to keep it under their control. I can deal with that now. The reality says that is does exist and my spirituality says that it doesn't have to. He also referred me to a cardiologist and a neurologist. I was later referred to a neurology specialist in multiple sclerosis at the University of Pennsylvania Medical Center. That was Dr. Kolson, a Penn State alumnus. We both attended Penn State at the same time in the 1970's. He didn't know me as William Hutton when I first met him, but when I said they called me by my nickname, Neil, he knew right away who I was.

Most of the test results were not much of a surprise to me. I knew of the things that were physically wrong over the years; the sports related injuries, the blood pressure, the heart murmur, and the herniated disks. I didn't know of the extensive nerve damage in my legs or that my heart valve would need to be fixed, or that there were white spots on my brain. This is why I didn't want to go to the doctor, but it is also why I'm glad I did.

There is one thing that happened recently that used to happen in the past, which I had completely forgotten about. I even forgot to tell my neurologist. I will tell him at my next appointment. Every few months I get a tender spot in the top of my head. This spot is very sensitive and I cannot put any pressure on it. The tenderness lasts for about a day. I used to think it was because I would bump the top of my head periodically in the attic. But the tenderness wouldn't come immediately after the bump. It may not happen until weeks or months after the bumping and it wouldn't necessarily be in the same spot that I bumped. Whether or not this has something to do with MS, I don't know. It was just another thing to think about.

When I went to Dr. Kolson for my second visit and a review of my test results, he had a resident doctor with him. I know that he was there to learn and observe, but somewhere in the back of my mind, I felt that he could have been there to help restrain me if I went ballistic at the results. At the end of my first visit with Dr.

Kolson, he said that he thought that I might have MS, but he was not permitted to give a positive diagnosis until all of my tests were completed. Based on my previous test results, my episode history that I could recollect, and the fact that he had a patient who was a former athlete with the same type of episodes and history, he had formed a conclusion that was conclusive enough to briefly tell me about the different treatments for the disease.

When he gave me the diagnosis, I was in denial. I asked him if my blood pressure, herniated disks, and pinched nerve could cause what was happening. He said that my disks have caused nerve damage in my leg, but that was all. Everything couldn't be blamed on the things that I wanted. When he began to go into depth about the treatments, I did not want to hear about taking anymore medication. They were mostly injections. I did not like taking pills, let alone injections. I was thinking the whole time that I was going to let it play out. I was going to prove to them that I didn't have MS. I was going to wait until the next flare-up, officially known as an exacerbation. If it never came, then I was the one who was right. If it did come, I would take the medicine. I told the doctor that I would have to think about the treatments. I would let him know later when I was ready to begin. I really had no intention of beginning. I thought that way for approximately 4 hours.

When one has been positively diagnosed with MS, information about the disease and treatments are immediately given to read and review. Included in my information was a video of four people who had been diagnosed with MS. They were telling their story about living with the disease before and after the treatments. Each person was affected somewhat differently and was in various stages of the disease.

One person's story made me change my mind about the treatments. He had felt the same way I did about starting the medication. He was going to wait until the next exacerbation. But then he said, "If I knew then what I know now, I would have started the treatments right away." I was sold on starting the treatments. I called Dr. Kolson's office the next day to tell him I was ready to start taking Avonex because it was one injection per week. I could live with one injection per week because I was not afraid of needles and I didn't want to take any more pills than I absolutely had to.

My biggest concern with the medication was its proven effectiveness. There is no known medical cure for MS. Studies have shown that the medications can help to delay the occurrences of the exacerbation or slow down the degenerative process of the disease in some of the cases. But what would really be the progression of the disease if no medication were taken? It is impossible to figure. Is it better to be safe than sorry? That is what my final conclusion was based upon.

I am no longer the superman that I thought I was. I am just human like everyone else. I am subject physically to what other humans are subject to. My body had been able to resist a lot of things for a long time because of my physical, mental, and spiritual conditioning. I resisted colds, headaches, flu viruses and other sicknesses and diseases. I never gave time to dwelling on the negative, only the positive. That, in combination with my adrenaline and faith, kept me going. I couldn't take a rest because that was too human. I didn't want to be overcome by the toughness of life. I welcomed it as just something more that I had to do. Having Jesus in my life, made it bearable and doable.

KEEPING BUSY

During the 1990's, I maintained a very active lifestyle. I am a computer-programming consultant by trade. That, along with a wife and two athletically involved daughters, LaChan and Kori, alone would be enough for the average person to maintain. I also coached high school football, was the church administrator and director for a rapidly growing church, took care of my grandmother during her last few years of life and was a father figure to our adopted son, Ryan. I saw these responsibilities as just assignments that I had to fulfill as part of my calling as a husband, father, grandson, friend, leader, and mentor. Keeping up the pace never allowed me to succumb to anything that was happening physically to me during this time, although I did notice differences in my body.

There is one thing that I continually hear or read from doctors and those people diagnosed with MS and that is to stay active as much as possible. It is harder to fight the disease if you do nothing to challenge it, so staying active helps to do that. I believe that the human will is critical to the success of overcoming adversity. Combined with faith, it creates a bond that is stronger than any thing that can come against you. That's what my bible says, and I believe it.

I have other future projects to keep me busy including the development of a community center, assisting pastors with church building and development and more coaching. I am trying to remove stress from my life and environment, and one way is to cut back on my computer consulting to a part-time status. I would eventually like to replace it entirely with another source of income. The sooner, the better.

I began coaching football in the early 90's after being asked by Dave Riley to help him at Rancocas Valley High School. I had coached basketball at Burlington City High School with Bob Williams during the 80's and I enjoyed coaching at that level. Dave was a college opponent of mine who played for West Virginia University. After college, he played for the Philadelphia Stars, and then started coaching high school football.

When Dave stopped coaching to become the athletic director at Willingboro High School, I momentarily retired from coaching football. I eventually returned after being asked by my brother, Mark, who was the head coach of a new junior high unlimited weight team and then later was asked by Tyrone Belford to be the defensive coordinator for his Willingboro High School team. I accepted and we went on to win the County Football Championship and the number 2 ranking in South Jersey.

While I did all of this, I began to notice physical problems occurring increasingly. My legs were losing their strength, my eyes were having intermittent focusing problems, my toes and fingers were continually numb, and my stamina was diminishing. By this time, I had already been diagnosed with MS, but my treatment consisted of an all natural and diet based treatment. I was still in denial.

SEARCH FOR THE MISSING LINK

For years I have been talking to Beverly about the diseases and conditions that have been prevalent in our society over the last forty years. I have not done any research or gathered statistics, but I am a firm believer that our diets have contributed to our state of unhealthiness. As a result, we have become subject to more diseases, conditions, and more health problems.

Because we are an economically driven society, new and artificial products are constantly being created for our convenience and for profit, and as consumers, we continue to ingest all types of things that are not healthy and meant for our bodies. This includes our drinking water.

The pharmaceutical industry has exploded in size and worth to create products to treat almost anything and everything, but without curing power. That is because the curing power is not in the medicines or the operations, but it is within our own bodies. The problem is that we have not put our bodies in position to heal it, but have placed it in position to destroy itself or to be destroyed.

This brings me to my next step. I completely changed my diet to be an all natural and raw diet. I have taken medications, used doctors and chiropractors, exercised, increased my faith spiritually, prayed, fasted and changed my diet according to doctor specifications. After reading the testimonies of hundreds of others with previously incurable, degenerative, or just annoying diseases and conditions, and gathering nutritional information from my readings, the proper diet appears to be one of the answers for restoring the body back to its healthy state. It positions the body to become its own medicine for complete restored health. The testimonies have come from people who have completely recovered from cancer, tumors, arthritis, MS, herniated disks, high blood pressure, diabetes, schizophrenia, poor eyesight, heart conditions, and other diseases and conditions. By the time my book is published and distributed, I believe that my testimony will be one that can be added to the hundreds and thousands of others that have opened their eyes to freedom from disease, better health, and a longer, healthier life.

The book that my diet is based upon is called, "God's Way to Ultimate Health" written by Dr. George H. Malkmus with Michael Dye. I believe that it is a must read for anyone who would like to live a healthier life and not just accept the things that have been physically happening to our bodies for years. I have already begun telling people about the book after just a short time on the diet. I have noticed a significant change in my body already. My blood pressure right now is the best that it has ever been and I just started my diet six days ago. I have always regularly checked my pressure and noticed a significant lowering. At my doctor's appointment, the nurse and doctor both said that my blood pressure was perfect. That was never said before. I am sure that the medicine helps, but it never got it to the "perfect level" before. I am waiting to see what happens next. I am looking forward to a future without medicine.

The numbness in my fingers and toes also feels differently. The sheet and blanket lying on my toes at night no longer bothers me like it used to. It used to be so uncomfortable that I had to turn my feet sideways to sleep every night because the covers felt like a weight on my toes. I also feel more alert and don't require as much sleep as I used to. I get up early in the morning now and am ready to get started. My appetite has changed and I never get the urgency to have to eat anymore. I haven't been a big eater for a long time, so not eating was no big deal for me, but I did have an urgency to eat at certain times. Sometimes I will juice my vegetables if I don't feel like preparing a salad or have much time to sit down and eat. However, food preparation doesn't take much time anymore because I don't cook it. I mostly eat everything raw.

THE SCARE

On Monday, May 7th, I woke up as usual and went downstairs to prepare for my weekly injection. It takes a couple of minutes for me to prepare the injection and then Beverly comes down to administer it into my thigh muscle. Fifteen minutes before the injection I would take 2 Tylenol capsules to lessen the side effects of the medication. I had never experienced any side effects of the medication from the day that I started the medication on March 12, of the previous year. I receive regular monthly check-up calls from counselors to monitor my progress with the medication. Each time the caller would be ecstatic that I had never experienced any side effects.

Side effects appeared to be a big concern of the Avonex medication. The effects are flu-like symptoms including chills, muscle aches, headaches, fever, etc. Many people experience the side effects because the body requires time to adjust to the concentrated influx of protein (in this particular case, interferon beta) into their system. This drug stimulates the production of immune system chemicals. The duration of the side effects is different for everyone. They can last from hours to days to weeks. I had never experienced any noticeable side effects. I originally told my counselors that I wasn't worried about the side effects and that I would probably experience the minimal. I knew my body at least to some degree.

Because I was doing so well with the medication, prior to my previous weekly injection I purposely did not take the Tylenol. I still did not experience any side effects after the injection. I always maintained the goal for years that I would minimally take medication, no matter what reason. I did not just take medication because I had a cold or headache or some other ailment. I always tried to give my body time to take care of the situation. I was following my normal plan of action with eliminating the Tylenol. What I didn't take into account was that I had just started a new diet and it was changing my body. My body wasn't necessarily going to react the same way to an injection of concentrated medication.

After the injection, I got on the computer to finish up some graphics work with LaChan that we were completing for our family reunion. Around lunchtime I told LaChan that I didn't feel well, that I had a slight headache and just general overall body ache. I told her that I was going to lie down for a few minutes expecting the feeling to just go away with rest. It didn't. It got worse.

I also realized that it was lunchtime and I had not eaten anything since my early morning carrot juice and barleygreen. So I went downstairs to get my normal fruit that I have for lunch. I noticed that I was having trouble with my balance and vision as well as the headache. My neck muscles also got very sore.

I brought the fruit upstairs, ate it, then proceeded to lie down on the bed and try to take a nap. It was a very restless nap. I noticed that my right hand and right leg were getting numb. Now I was really concerned. I had flashbacks of "the big one" last April. I thought I was having a relapse of MS. I called Beverly at her school and told her what was happening. She said she would come home right away. I also called Timmy to let him know. All I could think about was trying to start a new job and coaching having to fight through another long lasting episode of MS. I was angry.

Before Beverly got home, my father stopped by and Kori came home. We just sat around and talked. I could barely hold my head up because my neck was sore and it just felt more comfortable with it down. The fruit didn't help anything go away, although it didn't hurt anything. Eating was not the problem. The thing that I feared the most was what I thought was happening; my next exacerbation. I thought the medication was supposed to help prevent or postpone them. I was angry.

Beverly came home right after my Dad left. I was lying down again because it was too difficult to walk and my balance was off. I was concerned about the numbness on my right side. Beverly massaged my foot and leg. We began to talk about the disease. Why did it come back so soon? I couldn't wait for the diet to really kick in and begin restoring my body. I didn't realize at this moment that it had already begun.

I kept going over in my head what had I done differently. There were no significant changes since the previous week. I had just started the diet a few days before the previous injection; I didn't take the Tylenol that week and the injection went perfectly with no side effects. I maintained the diet up to this injection, I didn't take the Tylenol, the injection went perfectly and bam; it hit me. All the symptoms that I had were symptoms that were expected from my first injection of medication. My body was not the same after being on the diet for ten days. It reacted to the injection the way that was expected. I hadn't taken the Tylenol because I thought my body had adjusted to the medication. But now my body was different.

I knew before this, that my body was changing because of my blood pressure and numbness in my hands and feet, but under duress and pressure, sometimes we forget what we really know to be and just react to the situation. Sometimes that can be very dangerous but I knew that God would bring back to my remembrance what I needed because prayer was a constant in this entire episode.

I immediately limped into the bathroom to take 2 Tylenol capsules. Within one hour all of the symptoms were gone. What a relief. The diet is working and is changing my body. No matter what things appear to be, I know the real deal.

I have shared this information with people that I know who have incurable diseases or conditions, and with some that just want to get healthier and are serious about it. It is a process that will take some time. The amount of time depends upon the individual and the condition. God has given us the way. We must choose to accept it or reject it. Our biggest problem is trying to manipulate the way to our liking; taking an alternate route. We reap what we sow. That's scriptural.

MORE BUMPS

In the winter and early spring of 2004, I felt well enough to consider coaching again. I applied for the head football coaching job at my alma mater, Rancocas Valley Regional High School. I envisioned putting together an experienced proven staff, instilling character development principles, and using unfamiliar and new wave training techniques. I didn't foresee the losing of two of my major coaches, my rapid health decline and some other trouble spots along the way probably due to my lack of delegation. I asked for others to step up, but I didn't do a good enough job of transferring my thoughts and direction to the staff. The lack of physical strength had a direct influence on my mental capabilities.

Record wise, we were not successful, but we were on the verge of turning the corner...just a few plays away. The first year was experimental, but I knew what needed to be done the second year and opposing coaches saw it and encouraged me because they knew of my coaching ability as a defensive coordinator in the past. The problem was that after our year end banquet, my body shut down and I knew I was in trouble. I knew it was time to retire and that is what I did. I slept through the entire holiday season.

This eventually caused me to schedule appointments with my doctors, all three. The results were staggering to some degree, I was going through an MS exacerbation period (probably from the beginning of summer practice) and my heart valve needed immediate repair. The lack of adequate oxygen getting to my body was causing energy problems (as if the MS lack of energy problem wasn't enough).

So off I went into surgery on August 8, 2005. I was prepared physically, mentally, and spiritually. I couldn't wait to get my leaky valve fixed. It plagued me all of my football playing days. The doctors would always spend extra time listening to my heart but I would always pass my physical. I decided on a minimally invasive procedure by the best surgeon in the region for this type of surgery; Dr. Hargrove. The surgery went great and I was out of the hospital on the sixth day. My cardiac rehab went great also and I was back at work by November 1st.

There are many things that I began to learn about how MS affects Neil Hutton much differently than others with MS. First of all, I have no physical pain. Many MS patients have muscular pain and get treated for it. That has never been the case with me and it's a good thing. I have fought against medicines for years, so taking additional medicines was against my belief. It was recommended to me by my neurologist to replace the weekly Avonex injections with daily Copaxone injections and I began those on November 1, 2005. It is a daily subcutaneous injection. They are easy to take, but the thought of taking medicines forever which cannot cure is repulsive to me. So the first week in May 2006, I stopped the injections.

I was already taking blood pressure medication after the surgery and it was just a matter of time before my pressure came down and I would no longer need it. I thought about weaning myself from the Copaxone, but my demeanor was to do everything cold turkey and that is what I did. During May I felt a difference. I was able to sleep through the night from that point on. The anxiety of taking a shot and remembering where I took the last one every night was gone, but I began to have vision problems around mid May.

The first week in June the vision problems became too severe to drive so I began working from home. The problem with my eyes causes dizziness when walking and that affects my balance which is already shaky due to the MS. It makes it difficult to get around although I am okay sitting at the computer most of time. There were times of double vision for a couple of days, before I decided to give myself an injection. Low and behold, the next day my vision was slightly better. After one more injection the next day, my vision improved again.

After getting information from a holistic doctor, he said that the reaction I initially had was my body reacting to the lack of medicine. It was moving into exacerbation mode. Taking the injection was like a junkie needing a fix. The best thing was to wean myself away from the medicine and to not stop cold turkey. He said that I would probably feel better after the injection. I knew this was right and that was just the confirmation I needed.

So that is where I am today. I went to the eye doctor and he said no further damage has been done to my optic nerve and the focus issue is strictly MS related. That was good news. I am ready to consult with the holistic doctor and find a more natural way to combat this disease.

ADJUSTMENTS

The disease Multiple Sclerosis, has forced me to make many lifestyle adjustments. We purchased a boat (my hobby) in the fall after my heart surgery. It was Beverly's birthday present to me. We had one in the 80's and 90's, but had outgrown it for the purposes that we needed it for. We needed a larger boat for just relaxation, not recreation. I needed a stress relief, but did we get it?

We bought a 28 foot Bayliner with a kitchen, bathroom and 2 sleeping quarters from the father of one of my high school football players. He was moving away to Tennessee. We put it in the water in 2006 and took our first long trip in August to Cape May for a vacation. It was the best vacation week that we've ever had. Being on the water has always been special to me. Many of my sermons and ideas have come from being on or in the water. We are now in need of a larger boat to accommodate the grandchildren and their families. Thirty-eight to forty feet would suffice.

Although using the boat promotes relaxation, it requires normal routines to keep it maintained. As much as we like our boat, it is not optimum for my condition. Walking on the deck of the boat to reach the docking lines is very precarious. Usually I crawl through the windshield opening to the deck to reach the lines and sit while connecting or disconnecting them. Stretching to reach the side hose opening for the fresh water tank is also a major task. Because the boat rocks with the waves, standing during rocking can cause some balance issues. Climbing up to secure the window or canvas snaps involves securing oneself tightly with the free hand. These are activities done when the boat is docked. Just imagine the brain activity for decision making when the boat is moving.

The second adjustment we made was fixing the interior

of our house. That was a stress relief for Beverly. The bedrooms, kitchen, and living areas of the house were redone. It made her feel better and that also removed stress from me.

The third adjustment that I made was medically related. In 2007, I began steroid based treatments (ACTHAR GEL) to treat the symptoms of the MS. I never did that in the past but the symptoms now needed to be more controlled because it was getting increasingly difficult to hide them and it could become dangerous. That led me to the next adjustment.

The fourth adjustment made was to begin talking freely about the disease and what I have to go through each day. I had always kept that away from everyone except Beverly. Now I can explain what goes on inside my head when I have to do the simple things that everyone takes for granted. I never wanted anyone to feel sorry or have any pity on me, but people responded in a very accommodating way.

My body winds down in the evenings when I am not on the ACTHAR schedule. I lose strength in my legs and will use my cane if we have to be in close quarters or around a lot of people. The cane helps me to maintain my balance to keep from falling onto anyone or onto the floor. If we are sitting at a table anywhere, I try to not have to get up for any reason. In order to get up, I have to scan the entire room to find the easiest, least cumbersome path to where I have to go. I must check chair and body spacing, extended legs, and other obstacles that may interfere with my route. Any adjustment around or over an obstacle could create an unsteady balance issue.

The fifth adjustment has been my flexible work schedule. I have to incorporate all of my doctor appointments and blood tests into my calendar. I must also rest after taking my morning medications for a couple of hours which is why I don't usually go into the office until 9:30-10:00 am. If I took them at night, then I wouldn't be able to sleep through the night. That was discovered by trial and error. I usually stay at the office until after 6:00 pm and close the office. My cell phone number is always available to the office for emergencies, I can always login to the network from home, and I am only 7 minutes away if absolutely needed.

The sixth and maybe most critical adjustment to longevity and health has been the incorporation of chiropractic therapy into my lifestyle. Years ago I attended chiropractic sessions for back pain relief due to herniated disks, but the revelation that I now have of chiropractic care and its usefulness is beyond measure. Chiropractic care is not just for pain relief, but for promoting proper body self–healing. This is done by the realignment of vertebrae in order to maximize the proper nerve paths and blood flow in the body. This is what the body needs to heal itself. The body was been designed to be self-healing, but we don't maximize its greatest feature. This may be the missing link needed for complete restoration. That is what Burlington Chiropractic has taught me. I believe, along with God's guidance, that is the final piece of the puzzle. Thank you Burlington Chiropractic. I know that Montel Williams thanks you and all of the Chiropractic centers like yours. You will reap a great reward for your hearts toward people and their health.

THE MEMORY LAPSES

It is ironic how I forgot about this symptom of MS, but I may have been placing the blame on age instead of where it properly belonged. I have always been a detailed, logical, and organized thinker and planner, especially in my line of work as a computer programming consultant. Everything that we do is analyzed, designed, coded, and tested.

Under stressful situations, I can recall losing the ability to follow through on all of the steps required to complete a project. My mind knew the steps, but the large quantities of data being retained made me forget what I had completed and what I hadn't finished yet. Experience took away the need for logging every task, but that is not the case with MS. Years ago, I left one job with incomplete tasks for Y2K (unusual for me), but I didn't realize it until a new programmer came on board before I left and asked me about them. I realized my mistake when confronted, but it was too late for me to fix it and I apologized for the mishap. I explained the process for resolving it to them and left it for them to complete. I didn't want to leave a client in that manner but there was nothing more that could do. My contract had ended.

There have been a few other incidences with minor project slipups or physical mistakes. Some don't require immediate attention, but nonetheless, they were incorrect or incomplete at the time and eventually needed to be addressed. Now I try to always retrace my steps and thought process. Eventually I will fix the errors, but it leaves a blemish on my self-imposed reputation. I just have to do more thorough testing and retesting and can't just live with the first pass anymore. I can't trust my judgment 100%. Everything must be checked and rechecked, even with my close-up and peripheral vision. A few mishaps or close calls rekindles the fact that my judgment is impaired and cannot always be trusted.

This is the latest challenge that I have with Multiple Sclerosis. The mental and emotional issues have surpassed the physically imposed limitations. I can get immediate help with the physical things, but the other things play games with the mind. It is an ongoing battle that one must be willing to fight if you want to keep your sanity, confidence and productivity. I will not be overtaken by the disease because I still have too much to accomplish. I am moving into the area of experiencing the "passions of my heart". I cannot fully retire yet, I am too young to become a couch potato and card player.

I do miss playing golf and having sports workouts with the grandkids. I miss showing them what to do and don't like just telling them what to do. I will try to do selected activities this summer to help them apply what they have been learning and we'll see how it goes. My active time will be limited and recovery time is more valuable and necessary..

THE UNEXPECTED

As I mentioned in the previous chapter about life's stressful situations, for most of 2009, my condition remained fairly stable. However in July, there was a major change in the insurance carrier for my wife's benefits package. This meant that all of my medications were now covered through a different prescription plan and mail-order pharmacy. It wasn't a problem for my cardiology medications, but presented a problem for one of my MS medications, in particular the ACTHAR GEL. This was the every three month injections used to treat the recurring MS symptoms in order for me to live a suitable quality of life. The insurance company held up the approval of the medication for approximately two months, which meant that once approved or if approved, it would be about five months between treatments.

After appealing the denial, we made numerous visits to my neurologist and phone calls to state officials, celebrity acquaintances, insurance advocates and medical professionals. Holding down the stress levels became difficult and an MS exacerbation was beginning. I continued with my regular chiropractic visits which I believe helped me physically through this time. The appeal was accepted, the prescription was approved and the medication was delivered.

After five months of no injections, it was like starting all over again for my body. Drug side effects surfaced, the exacerbation process had already begun, and it took about two weeks for things to get back to somewhat normal, physically and emotionally. This was an unexpected roller coaster ride. Now it's time for a return to normalcy and consistency and to move on to a better more manageable life. MS is a challenge, but I have never avoided challenges and won't begin now. I am looking forward to rediscovering my lost golf game.

LIFE GOES ON

Through all of these setbacks, I have found it important to maintain a positive outlook and to continue to work within my limits. As a result of not being able to physically engage in the passions of my heart, such as coaching, I plan to stay involved as a consultant and mentor to the younger coaches and athletes (that is the reason for Reality Sports Group Inc.). I have experienced the growth and maturity of some of our former players, and heard from them regarding the impact that we had as coaches on their young adult lives. We are viewed as mentors, coaches and in some cases, fathers. I am proud to see them reach back in their growth to help younger kids along their way to maturity.

I now look at alternative careers choices through different eyes, based upon my abilities and disability, because I anticipate a long and prosperous future life. Included in our early retirement plans is the attaining of a law degree for myself, the anticipation of educational consulting opportunities for Beverly and possibly a move to South Africa or the Southern U.S. for business and climate reasons (to help with the MS). MS is not a reason for stopping or ending, but a reason for refocusing, readjusting and continuing.

Along the way I have become an ordained minister, a business consultant/owner, tax and will consultant, a notary, a sports camp director, as well as assuming other personal assistance consulting tasks. Prayerfully, the law degree will bring all of these things together. I expect that the post MS era will be greater than the pre MS era. God has a way of taking things that were meant for evil and turning them around to be used for our good.

Although I have been taking Acthar Gel treatments every three months, for the last two years, the Acthar Gel injections now seem to work for a shorter period of time. The injection treatments no longer last for the full three months, but are down to approximately two months. I can feel the lack of medication in my system during the last month of the three month cycle. When expressing this information to the doctor, he explained that the next step of treatment was using a much more powerful drug, similar to chemotherapy type drugs.

I told the doctor that a stronger drug was not an option. I would continue my current treatments and begin exercising more. I do feel better after exercising, so that might be the answer. So here I am, heading into the spring season with my next round of treatments to start in forty days, but exercising can begin immediately.

This is the part of MS that no one will understand, unless I tell them each step along the way, but I am not a complainer. They will know soon enough, especially when my mood swings begin. We laugh about it all the time and the girls will ask their mother, "What's wrong with Dad? " Then they are reminded. The toughest thing is to not become short-tempered with the grandkids. I will interact with them during that time doing fun things that they like to do.

The other tough part of dealing with MS is not letting life's stressful situations affect your life. The huge fuel oil tank leak that we had in January 2009 was a perfect example of that. In addition, our house was broken into and Beverly's jewelry was stolen. Those two major catastrophes could have initiated an exacerbation, but with the help of prayer, we saw this as a possible blessing and not a curse. The cleanup and removal of the oil in an environmentally sensitive area such as ours, was estimated to be as high as $50K. The results of the oil spill situation are now in the hands of our attorney. But our faith in God has enabled us to endure during this time of trouble and anticipation. We thank God that the MS symptoms have remained under control. Now what's around the corner?

Made in the USA
Charleston, SC
02 February 2012